GREG AMUNDSON

THE WARRIOR

A FABLE ABOUT

AND

FULFILLING YOUR POTENTIAL

THE MONK

AND FINDING TRUE HAPPINESS

THE WARRIOR AND THE MONK

A FABLE ABOUT FULFILLING YOUR POTENTIAL AND FINDING TRUE HAPPINESS

First Edition

ISBN: 978-1-61170-272-9

By Greg Amundson
3703 Portola Drive, Santa Cruz, CA 95060
www.GregoryAmundson.com

Edited by Patricia Bond

Book Design by Brooktown Design, www.brooktown.com

Illustrations by Joseph Carlos Fitzjarrell, www.fitznice.com

Legal Disclaimer by the Author:
The characters "Young Warrior," "Wise Monk," and many of the other characters, events and places appearing in this work and their names are fictitious and were created by the author's imagination. Any resemblance to real persons, living or dead, is purely coincidental. Bible references are in bold and may be found in the New King James Bible. The term, "Ancient Prophet," refers collectively to the Prophets of the Old Testament. The term, "Greatest Prophet," refers to our Lord Jesus Christ. This work is not meant to treat or cure any mental health condition. Persons experiencing any form of mental or emotional health condition to include PTS or MST are encouraged to seek the professional counseling of a licensed, qualified physician, therapist, or other competent professional.

Published by: **Robertson Publishing**™
www.RobertsonPublishing.com

PRAISE FOR THE WORK OF GREG AMUNDSON

"I often tell people at my seminars, 'We don't need more Buddhists in the world, we need more Buddhas. We don't need more Christians, we need more Christ-like beings.' And such is the case with my amazing, breathing brother Greg Amundson. He's not one of those wishy-washy, praise the Lord, in-your-face, superficial Christians: He is a former SWAT Operator, DEA Special Agent, U.S. Army Captain, and CrossFit athlete and coach. He is a spiritual warrior, and he carries God in his heart. His book, *The Warrior and the Monk,* is one of those books you can open and find pure inspiration." – *Dan Brulé,* world renowned lecturer and international best selling author of *Just Breath*

"Sometimes our mythic roots carry the most powerful insights, and Greg Amundson's new fable, *The Warrior and the Monk,* is no exception. Greg leverages his remarkable storytelling ability to help the reader acquire new insights that serve to strengthen the spiritual core. Wisdom is waiting to be discovered in *The Warrior and the Monk*—a must-read for strengthening the mind, body, and spirit." – *Josh Mantz,* Former Army Major and #1 Amazon bestselling author of *The Beauty of a Darker Soul*

"Greg fought the war on drugs, battled in the streets, on behalf of our nation. Now he fights to inspire us to overcome our fears, flaws and failures, battling for the glory of God. Pick up *God In Me* and *The Warrior and the Monk* and let God's work, through Greg's words and stories, uplift your mind, body and soul." – *Jay Dobyns,* author of *New York Times* bestseller *No Angel,* and *Catching Hell*

"Greg's ability to transcend boundaries and speak to the essence of spirituality is profound and encouraging. East meets West here in a beautiful union of human experience, discipline, and philosophy. By following the timeless advice in Greg's new book, *The Warrior and the Monk*, we can happily discover that what we are searching for has been within us the entire time." – *Scott McEwen,* #1 *New York Times* bestselling co-author of *American Sniper;* national bestselling *Sniper Elite Series,* and the new *Camp Valor* series of novels

"Greg Amundson's book, *The Warrior and the Monk,* makes experiencing God a little more accessible. It is a great primer for the new seeker and wonderful refresher for the seasoned traveler." – *Rev. Deborah L. Johnson,* author of *The Sacred Yes* and *Your Deepest Intent*

"Greg Amundson's expert instruction has brought dramatically greater strength, balance, and vital energy into my daily life as it has the lives of countless others. Now, with *The Warrior and the Monk*, Greg guides us in channeling that newfound strength and energy toward a life of service, love, wisdom, and true fulfillment. A powerful and transformational book that will inspire you to live your very best life." – *Girish*, musician, teacher, and author of *Music and Mantras: The Yoga of Mindful Singing for Health, Happiness, Peace and Prosperity*

"Greg Amundson's groundbreaking new title, *The Warrior and the Monk*, is an inspiring, timely and courageously articulated perspective on seeking (and discovering) a personal relationship with God." – *Robert Vera*, author of #1 Amazon bestseller, *A Warrior's Faith*, and founder of the Eagle Rise Speakers Bureau

"Greg's books, *God In Me* and *The Warrior and the Monk*, capture in words the epic quest we are all on to find happiness, meaning, and fulfillment in life. Greg articulates in a groundbreaking ministry that by turning our attention inward, and seeking God, we can find purpose in our life, and joy through being of service to others." – *Karen Vaughn*, Gold Star mother of US Navy SEAL Aaron Carson Vaughn, and bestselling author of *World Changer: A Mother's Story*

"Greg Amundson IS a Modern Day WARRIOR MONK. Greg has lived it, serving as both an army officer, DEA Special Agent and SWAT Operator, and in his daily training program to maintain the warrior mind and body that helped create the CrossFit movement of elite tactical fitness. As both a warrior and Christian, I can attest that Greg's new book brings all these facets of life together and articulates them in a groundbreaking fashion. If you are Christ follower and a man or woman aspiring to live the warrior ethos, I highly recommend this book." – *Jason Redman*, US Navy SEAL (Retired), founder of the Combat Wounded Coalition, and author of *The Trident – The Forging and Reforging of a Navy SEAL Leader*

"Greg is the epitome of the way we all should strive to be better each and every day. With grace, joy and a powerful passion to help others, he instills in all of us the beauty of life and the importance of following God. His books, *God In Me* and *The Warrior and the Monk*, will help you along your own path of self-discovery and reveal just how important you are in making this world a better place." – *Kevin R. Briggs*, Sergeant, California Highway Patrol (Retired), and author of *Guardian of the Golden Gate, Protecting the Line Between Hope and Despair*

"Greg Amundson is a warrior with a monk-like mindset. His own self discovery and passion to help others is truly inspiring. Greg empowers us with the tools to a disciplined mind, spirituality and perfect work-life balance." – *Dr. Suhas Kshirsagar BAMS, MD(Ayu)*, author of #1 Amazon bestseller, *Change Your Schedule Change Your Life*

ALSO BY GREG AMUNDSON

Published Books

Firebreather Fitness – Work your Mind, Body and Spirit into the Best Shape of your Life (Velo Press – 2017)

God In Me – Daily Devotionals for a Heart like Christ (Robertson Publishing – 2016)

Your Wife is NOT Your Sister – And 15 Other Love Lessons I Learned the Hard Way (Robertson Publishing – 2013)

CrossFit Journal Articles®

A Chink in My Armor

Coaching the Mental Side of CrossFit

CrossFit Headquarters—2851 Research Park Drive, Santa Cruz, CA

Diet Secrets of the Tupperware Man Vol. I

Diet Secrets of the Tupperware Man Vol. II

Forging Elite Leadership

Good Housekeeping Matters

How to Grow a Successful Garage Gym

Training Two Miles to Run 100

CrossFit Goal Setting Work Book

Social Media

The Greg Amundson Show on iTunes (Podcast)

YouTube.com/AmundsonGreg

ACKNOWLEDGEMENTS

First and foremost, I am deeply grateful for the everlasting love and embrace of God and His Son, Jesus Christ. For my beloved parents, Raymond and Julianne Amundson, who encouraged me from a young age to develop my mind, body, and spirit in such a manner that I could be of greater service to others. A great deal of appreciation is extended to Brooklyn Taylor for her brilliant layout and design contributions to this book, and to Joe Fitzjarrell for bringing the characters and scenes to life in his drawings. I am also indebted to the plank owners of the Patriot Authors Network and Eagle Rise Speakers Bureau: Robert Vera, Josh Mantz, Jay Dobyns, Jason Redman, Kevin Briggs, and Karen Vaughn. Your true "Warrior Monk" spirit continues to inspire me more every day. Special thanks to Joe De Sena and my dear friend, TJ Murphy, of SPARTAN, for believing in this project and contributing to the foreword of this book. Finally, to the great mentors and masters whose leadership has deeply influenced my life: Rev. Deborah L. Johnson, Mark Divine, Dan Brulé, Londale Theus, Ken Gray, Chaplain Richard Johnson, Pastor Dave Hicks, Dr. Deepak Chopra, Dr. Suhas Kshirsagar, Raja John Bright, Maharishi Mahesh Yogi, Baba Hari Dass, and Pastor René Schlaepfer.

THE WARRIOR
AND THE MONK

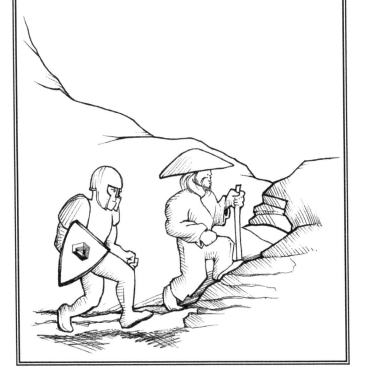

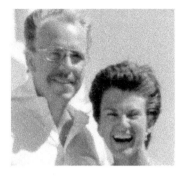

This book is dedicated in loving memory to
my mom and dad, the greatest "Warrior Monks"
I have ever known.

———

"God is more worthy of your pursuit,
attention, and love than all the other passions
of the world combined."
— *Dr. Raymond Amundson*

———

"God is entirely devoted to your advancement."
— *Julianne Amundson*

CONTENTS

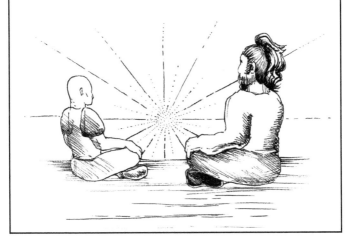

SPARTAN UP!

"You can join the movement toward a life of service, discipline and exhausting, exhilarating effort. It's not the good life. It's the best life. And we need you."

— Joe De Sena

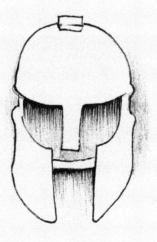

Greg Amundson is many things: a public servant, a coach, a teacher, a fitness pioneer, and through it all, a Warrior. A "True Warrior" who dedicates his life to self-mastery in service of others.

Greg was a young man when he made the commitment to be a Warrior who serves others. He knew it was a life-long commitment. He knew it had nothing to do with a time clock he punched in and out of; it was every hour of every day. He finished a night shift as a cop, then attended the first workout of the day at the original Cross-Fit gym in Santa Cruz, CA.

That workout was one discipline of many. He trained his body, his mind, and his spirit. He abstained from alcohol and started each day with a ritualistic approach to hard exercise and mindfulness. Results weren't left to chance; he became the best at what he did.

Lives depended on how well Greg executed his duties. Every degree of performance mattered, so he aggressively pursued improvement with an enthusiastic disdain for mediocrity.

Greg applied this work ethic toward serving as a Deputy Sheriff on a SWAT Team, then as a DEA Special Agent and Captain in the U.S. Army. When he was not protecting and serving on the street, Greg was teaching CrossFit movement and theory, spending his weekends educating people of all walks of life how to "get comfortable with the uncomfortable" and be prepared for "the unknown and the unknowable."

This included being one of the founding leaders of the CrossFit movement and his relentless encouragement for including constantly varied, functional movement at high intensity (CrossFit) within the law enforcement profession.

The role of a leader is to help people help themselves. This is Greg's modus operandi. As they say, give a man a fish. When Greg teaches, he is not only doing that but providing tools that can be used to succeed, and the inspiration for using each one along the way.

Plus, if necessary, a push.

But along with the push, Greg knows how important it is to teach a beginner what it feels like to succeed. This is what provides the energy and excitement that will drive the student toward learning and self-mastery and eventually completely transforming their life. Greg understands the importance of developing the mind, body, and spirit, and he strikes the perfect balance between the complementary worlds of the Warrior and the Monk.

I believe Greg would have felt at home in the early days of Spartan. It was seventeen years ago. I had left Wall Street with one goal in mind: to change 100 million lives by motivating people to get out of their comfort zone and embrace a Warrior lifestyle.

Spartan was forged from grit around our kitchen table after long morning hikes, carrying rocks up mountains. In 2018, we now have 200 races in 30 countries and three million people living the Spartan way.

Greg and I share the same desire to spread the message about how to bring meaning, purpose and discipline to one's life; to not only make one's own life better, but also to improve their community and the world.

As a global community, we face many daunting and seemingly overwhelming challenges. What can you as a single person do?

You can join the movement toward a life of service, discipline, and exhausting, exhilarating effort. It's not the good life. It's the best life. And we need you.

And the first step is reading the book, *The Warrior and the Monk,* and considering the "Way of the Warrior" as Greg Amundson is now teaching it.

Hope to see you out there fighting your way up a mountain. I'll be joining you.

  — *JOE DE SENA*

SPARTAN Founder & CEO and #1 *New York Times* bestselling author of *Spartan Up! A Take-No-Prisoners Guide to Overcoming Obstacles and Achieving Peak Performance in Life* and *Spartan Fit! 30 Days. Transform Your Mind. Transform Your Body. Commit to Grit.*

PART ONE

THE YOUNG WARRIOR

"A true warrior is one who masters themselves

to be of greater service to the world."

— The Wise Monk

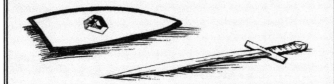

Once there was a young warrior . . .

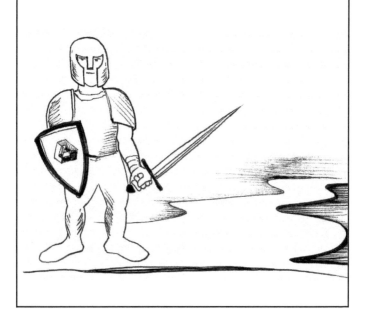

Who carried a sword and a shield. He pursued treasure and the dragons of the earth, and relished in the accolade of his accomplishments.

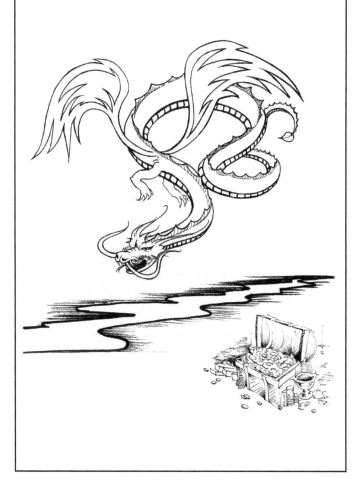

However, the more the young warrior

Acquired

Achieved and

Aspired to...

The greater was his sense of

Poverty

Lack and

Purposelessness.

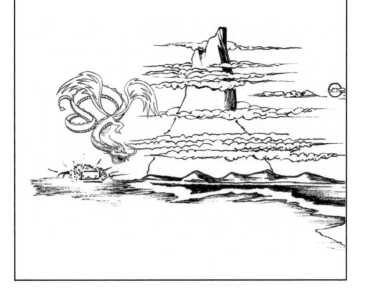

So the young warrior sought out the counsel of an old monk, the wisest person he knew. And thus, unbeknownst to the young warrior, he embarked upon....

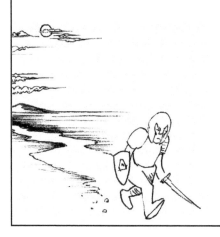

A quest to find God.

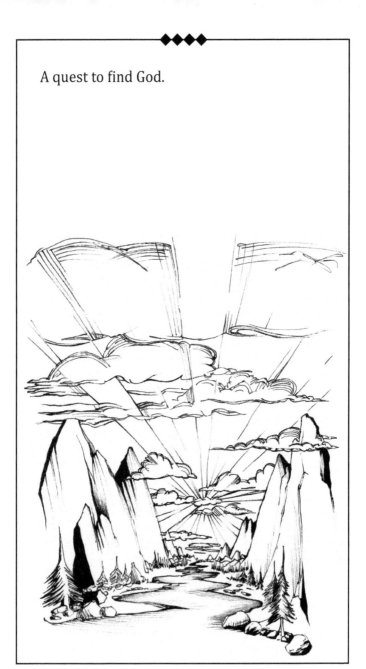

PART TWO

THE WISE MONK

"The river of God is always

running through you."

— The Wise Monk

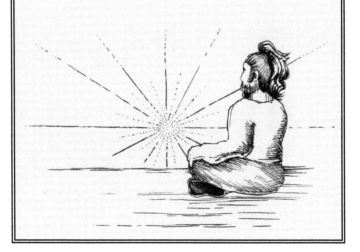

Many years ago...

The wise monk had also lived as a young warrior. At that time, no amount of worldly treasure was enough to satisfy his desires, and he fell into a great depression.

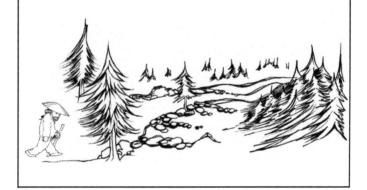

In much despair

he

e m b a r k e d

upon...

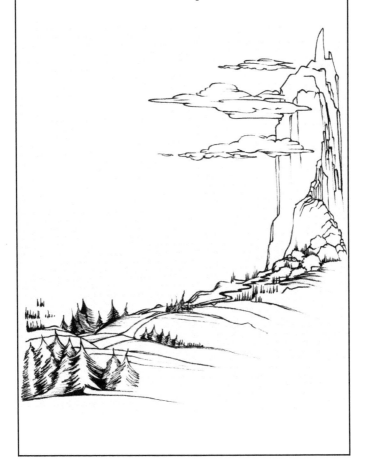

A quest to find God.

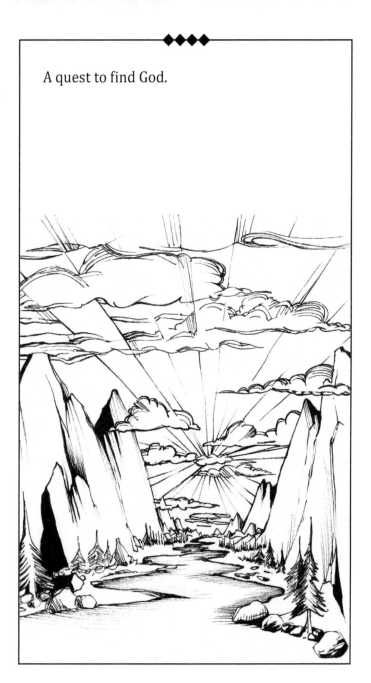

Casting aside all he had worked so hard to acquire, the wise monk began in earnest upon his quest.

He relentlessly searched

across the farthest corners of the earth...

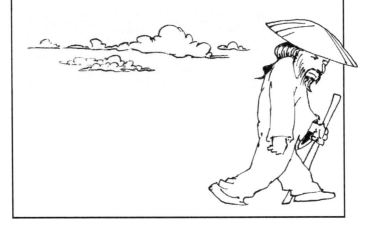

He   subjected   himself   to   the   most
extreme of ordeals...

And felt certain that God would surely reveal
Himself upon the peak of the next mountain.

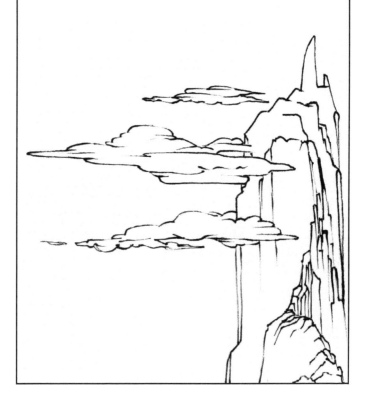

However...

the **harder**

further

and

l o n g e r

he searched for God, the greater distance he felt he still needed to go.

It seemed to the wise monk that he would never find God.

Then one day, it suddenly occurred to the wise monk...

Perhaps he was searching in the

wrong
d i r e c t i o n.

And so the wise monk sat down, took a deep breath, and became still.

And much to his surprise...

The wise monk found that in the stillness of his mind, God had been waiting for him the entire time.

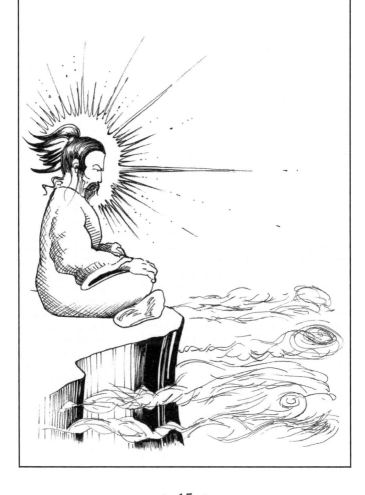

PART THREE

THE JOURNEY WITHIN

"The source of your desire is already

within you."

— The Wise Monk

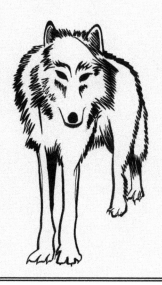

"How can I **find happiness?**" the young warrior asked the wise monk.

"Everything **I work so hard to achieve,** thinking that it will make me happy, **soon loses** its attractiveness."

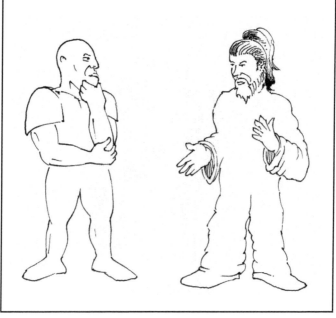

"Perhaps it is because you consider

happiness and
	attractiveness to be the
same thing," replied the wise monk.

Then the wise monk said,

"You were not created to find
	lasting happiness from
	the objects, conditions, or treasures of the
outer world."

Startled and amazed by what he heard, the young warrior quietly knelt down before the wise monk. The young warrior knew he was in the presence of someone who had acquired great wisdom.

The wise monk explained,

"Because you **project** your awareness into the world of **material objects,** you focus on the creation, instead of the **Creator."**[1]

After a shared moment of silence, the wise monk said,

"In other words, you have spent your life focusing on treasure. The key is to **refocus** your **attention** on the **Supreme Source** of treasure."

"Consider a dehydrated man attempting to quench his thirst by sipping dew from a small blade of grass," proposed the wise monk.

"That would be foolish," the young warrior replied, "For his thirst would never be fully satisfied."

"You are exactly right," the wise monk said encouragingly.

Then the wise monk continued,

"If only the dehydrated man knew there was an

unbounded

unlimited

and

infinitely abundant

reservoir of water he could drink from. Then his thirst would be

forever fulfilled."

"Now consider this," said the wise monk…

"Would it make sense for the dehydrated man to fill up containers of water, to hoard them, bury them, protect them, or possess over them?"

The young warrior thought for a moment, and then replied,

"Certainly not. For anytime the man was thirsty, he could simply return to the reservoir, and drink all the water he wanted."

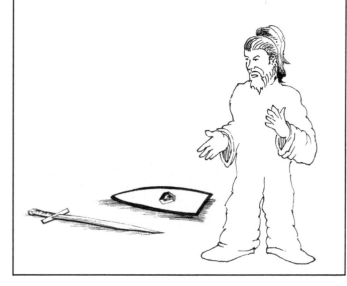

"Once again, you are exactly right. You see, young warrior, much of the wisdom you seek is already within you."

Then the wise monk explained a key insight for the young warrior to contemplate.

"The metaphor of the dehydrated man teaches a very important lesson. The blade of grass represents treasure, while the abundant reservoir of water represents the **source of treasure.**

Only the source was able to quench the man's thirst...

"And furthermore, the **source was always available to the man.** He could drink from the source anytime he desired.

Now imagine if the **abundant reservoir** of water **was already within you,"** said the wise monk.

"If that were the case, I would never be thirsty again," answered the young warrior.

The young warrior pondered this insight for a moment, and then thought to himself,

"Perhaps this story of the dehydrated man is about me. It seems I have been trying to fill myself from the outside in, instead of from the inside out. Could it be possible that the source of everything I have been searching for is already within me?"

The young warrior felt increasingly inspired and encouraged in his quest to find happiness. A part of the young warrior felt the wise monk was teaching him a storehouse of new information...

While simultaneously, another part of the young warrior felt he was simply being reminded of something he knew long ago.

PART FOUR

THE CAUSE
OF EFFECTS

"The cause of the effects in your life

are your thoughts."

— The Wise Monk

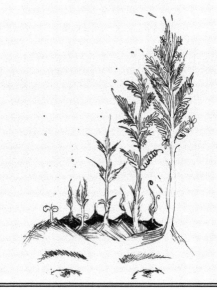

The wise monk happily recognized the twinkle of awakening in the young warrior's eyes. Continuing his discourse, the wise monk remarked,

"Most people concern themselves with external things. They give their attention almost exclusively to the outer world, thinking the world will fulfill their desires.

However, these people are greatly deceived because...

They think that source and treasure are the same thing.

And they also...

Mistakenly believe that cause and effect are the same thing as well."

The young warrior listened intently as the wise monk opened his mind to a new way of perceiving the world.

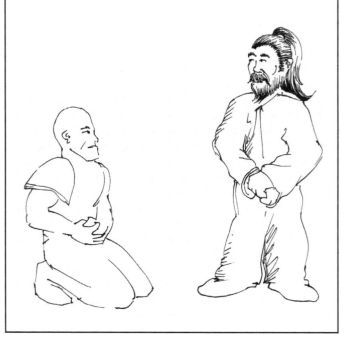

Then the wise monk continued,

"This was how I viewed the world for many years. Then one day, in a moment of **peaceful stillness** and **silence,** I realized something profound."

Looking deeply into the eyes of the young warrior, the wise monk said,

"I discovered the **outer world** was but the **final outcome**

that was **created within my mind."**

"The cause was within me; the effect was therefore outside of me.

In order to change the effects of my life,

I first needed to change their cause."

The young warrior then asked a very important question,

"What was the *cause* of the *effects* of your life?"

The wise monk answered, "It is the same for every person in the entire world...

The cause of effects

are

your

thoughts."

"Do you mean my **thoughts create things?**" The young warrior asked with a startled expression on his face.

"That is correct," said the wise monk, who then continued...

"And for this reason, the ancient Prophets said,

'As a man thinketh in his heart, so is he.'[2]

All warriors must therefore guard their heart with vigilance,

'For out of the heart are all matters of life.'"[3]

The wise monk then reflected,

"You see, although I now walk the path of a monk, at one time in my life, I was a warrior, and as a warrior, I pursued with a vengeance dragons and the treasures of the world."

"Did you carry a sword and shield?" asked the young warrior.

"Yes, and like you, my sword and shield were put to use exclusively in the world of *effects*."

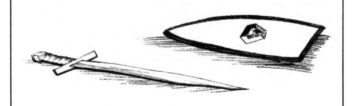

The wise monk paused for a moment to ensure the young warrior was listening intently, and then said,

"But soon I realized the greatest use of my sword and shield would be to

serve and protect
the world of cause."

Through the use of an ancient parable, the wise monk then continued to elaborate on the nature of thoughts, and their relationship with the effects of the world.

"Young warrior, listen carefully, for the lesson contained within this story is exceedingly important for you to understand...

"Many years ago, an old sage spoke to a young boy on the evening before he would begin the ritual inauguration into the warrior tradition. The young boy was apprehensive and uncertain of his ability to succeed in the harsh training and conditions that would follow.

The old sage told the young boy,

"There are two wolves engaged in a fierce battle within your mind:

A Wolf of Courage

and...

A Wolf of Fear."

The young boy asked the old sage,

"Which wolf will be victorious in the battle?"

"Whichever wolf you feed," the old sage replied.

"In that case," the young boy thought aloud...

"I must feed the Wolf of Courage."

The old sage then said something that forever shaped the young boy's maturity into the warrior culture...

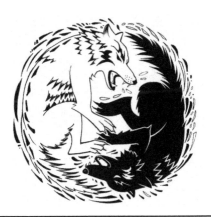

'The Wolf of Courage and the Wolf of Fear are both starving for your **attention,** which is **governed** by your **thoughts** and **words.**

A warrior must have...

discipline and **willpower** to

think and **speak** **positively.**

Only **positive** thoughts and words shall feed the Wolf of Courage."

Hearing this ancient story retold by the wise monk elated the young warrior and captured his imagination. The story also sparked his interest in the power of not only thoughts, but of words as well.

"Wise monk, in the story you said the Wolf of Courage was fed by both thoughts and words. What effect does my speaking have in the world of effects?"

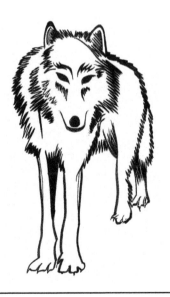

The wise monk replied,

"Your **speaking** is the
first effect of your thinking.

Every word you speak creates a ripple

throughout the entire Universe.

Your **speaking influences
your actions,** and over time and

with repetition, your **actions
shape** the **person** you **become."**

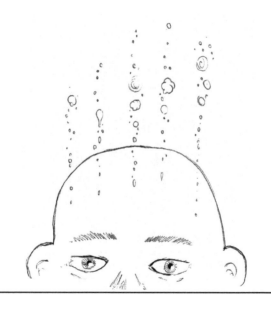

With a startled expression on his face, the young warrior exclaimed,

"I had no idea my thoughts and words were so powerful!"

"Indeed, young warrior..."

the wise monk said,

"They are the seeds you plant in the fertile soil of pure potentiality."(4)

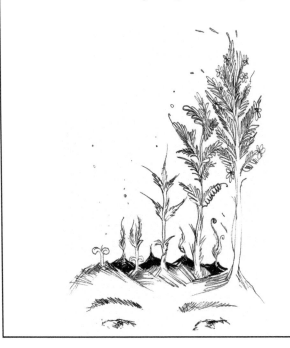

In order to help the young warrior understand the magnitude of power his thoughts and words contained, the wise monk said,

"A farmer who plants an apple seed is not surprised when an apple tree begins to grow, for the apple seed produced after its own kind. In the same manner, your words produce like seeds. Everything you say takes on life, and in time, everything you say will be returned to you in some way, shape, or form."[5]

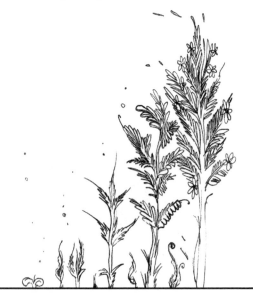

Hearing this, the young warrior asked,

"Is this why I must discipline my thinking?"

The wise monk said with encouragement,

"Yes, that is correct.

Your thinking is the point of inception

for everything you speak. Therefore, by disciplining your thinking, you begin to

speak a language of positive expectancy."

The wise monk then gently put his hands on the young warrior's shoulders, and said,

"Remember this sequence of events, and you can assure yourself a future of prosperity, love and fulfillment...

Positive thoughts
lead to positive words,

which produce after their kind, resulting

in positive experiences

within every area of your life."

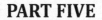

PART FIVE

FINDING THE
TRUE SOURCE

"Your True Source of strength is the

presence of God within you."

— The Wise Monk

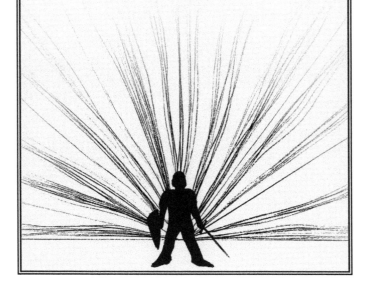

The wise monk and young warrior held eye contact for several moments, and then the wise monk said something very profound...

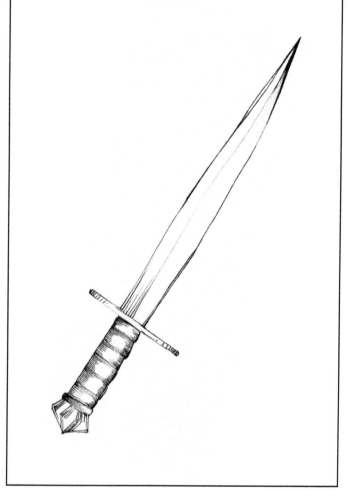

"When you use your sword to cut out of your mind all forms of negativity, and your shield to guard against the illusion of separateness from the desires of your heart, then you will faithfully understand the path of a true warrior."

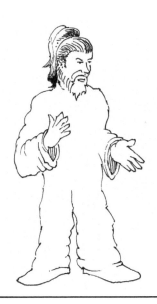

"What is a true warrior?" asked the young warrior.

"A true warrior is one who masters themself to be of greater service to others,"

answered the wise monk, who then continued,

"And in order to master yourself, you must develop a personal relationship with your True Source of strength."

"And where do I find my True Source?" the young warrior asked.

"Your True Source of strength is the presence of God within you," replied the wise monk.[6]

Startled, the young warrior asked,

"You mean, God is within me?"

"Yes, indeed!" the wise monk replied with a smile on his face. "And because the **presence** of God is **within** you, and **God** is the **Source** of **everything** you desire, when you embark on the quest to find God, you happily discover that everything you have been...

searching for

and **fighting** for

and **struggling** for

and **longing** for

and **working** for...

"Has been

within you

the entire time."[7]

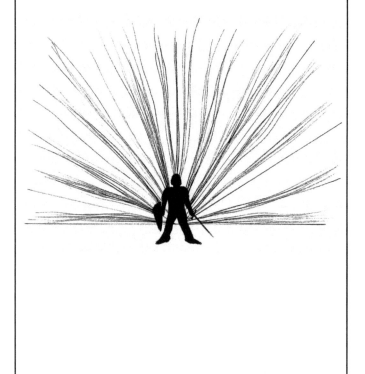

Overjoyed with a sense of increased self-realization, the young warrior became eager to start the quest to find his **True Source** of strength.

Thanking the wise monk for his mentorship and kindness, the young warrior stood up in preparation to depart.

The wise monk remarked,

"Remember, young warrior, on the journey you now embark upon, that your effort will never go to waste.

Even a **little progress** on the path of knowing your **True Source** will be of **immense value.**"[8]

PART SIX

THE DRAGONS

"It has been said, 'Your ego will

deceive you by edging God out.

E–G–O = Edge God Out.'"

— The Wise Monk

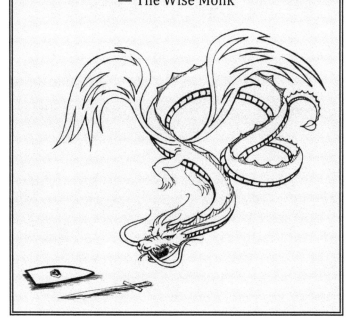

For several months, the young warrior was happy. He remembered the words of the wise monk, and was grateful for the knowledge he had gained during their time together.

However...

The young warrior sometimes wondered,

"Could it be, that my thoughts really create the conditions and experiences of my life?"

This notion began to frustrate the young warrior.

"If this were the case, I would be accountable to my thoughts, and how can I possibly control my thinking?"

Believing this to be impossible, the young warrior focused on the outer conditions of the world rather than the inner conditions of his mind.

And soon enough, the young warrior returned to what he knew best. He focused on dragons, and on acquiring the treasures of the world.

Yet it seemed to the young warrior the more he focused on dragons, the more dragons appeared within the conditions of his life.

And the more the young warrior focused on acquiring treasure, the more treasure he still wanted to have.

Sadly, it never occurred to the young warrior that everything he focused his attention on was increasing in his life. If only the young warrior was able to focus his attention on his True Source...

And in due time, the young warrior's **constant focus on dragons and treasure,** turned the young warrior into...

A dragon obsessed with treasure.

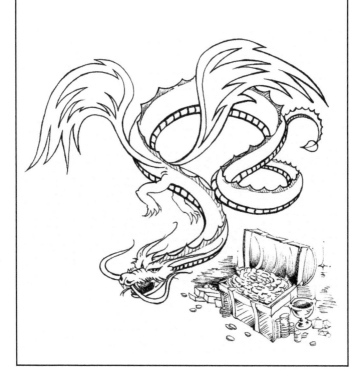

The young warrior's **ego** had him convinced that he *was* the possessions and **treasures** he had acquired...

And that he was what he did...

And that he was what other people thought of him...

And that he was separate from everybody else...

And that he was separate from what he felt was missing in his life.

And worst of all,

His ego had edged God out.

The young warrior had become consumed with the world of effects. And sadly, the young warrior had forgotten a key lesson the wise monk had instructed:

"Effects are the final outcome. In order to **experience new effects,** you must **change their root cause.**

The cause of your effects,

Is

Your

Thinking."

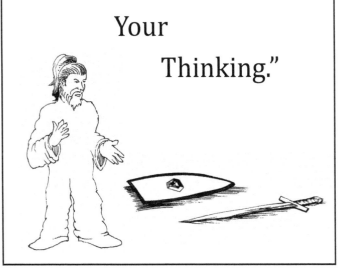

Soon the young warrior's **thinking** **became very negative,**

and therefore the **conditions** of his life...

became **very dark,** indeed.

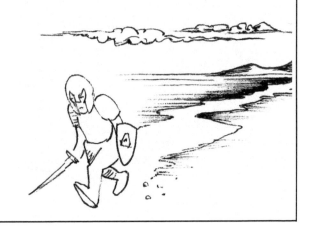

Regrettably, the young warrior had forgotten the **real dragons** he was fighting,

and the **real treasure** he was searching for...

Were both to be **found within**.

Finally, in despair and resignation, the young warrior returned to the counsel of the wise monk.

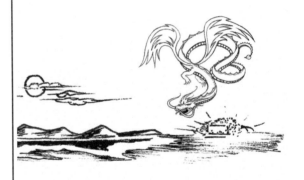

PART SEVEN

CHILD OF GOD

"Happiness is not something you can find. Happiness is what you are when you remember who you are."

— The Wise Monk

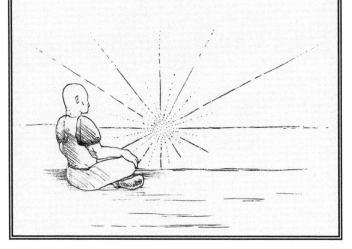

The wise monk immediately recognized the young warrior approaching, and went forward to greet him.

"Welcome young warrior! Why the look of defeat upon your face today?" the wise monk inquired.

With a great sigh of sorrow, the young warrior answered,

"I am worse off than the last time I saw you. Everything I have worked so hard to achieve has failed me."

The young warrior once again knelt down before the wise monk and said,

"Monk, I know that you are very wise, and I come to you for help in my quest to find true happiness."

The wise monk replied,

"Before we talk about happiness, I have one question for you...

"Who are you?"

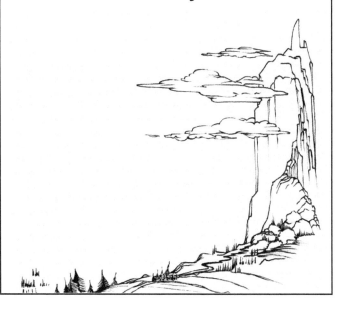

The young warrior thought to himself,

"What a silly question, I know exactly who I am."

With a hint of irritation in his voice and a **stirring of ego** within his mind, the young warrior added,

"I am a warrior, of course."

Then the young warrior **elaborated quite extensively** on a long list of his **accomplishments, achievements, positions held,** and of course, the **prized treasures** he worked so hard to accumulate. The young warrior also spoke for what seemed an eternity about the **dragons** he faced, and the **injustices** he had experienced throughout his life.

All the while, the wise monk listened attentively, without making a sound.

When the young warrior finally stopped speaking, the wise monk said,

"Very well, but I still have one question for you...

"Who are you?"

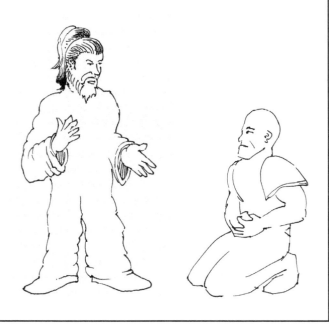

"What do you mean, 'Who am I?'" exclaimed the young warrior. "I just told you!"

The wise monk calmly replied,

"No, you did not. You told me your name. You told me your profession. You told me the things you've done. You told me about what other people say you are.

You told me about the titles you achieved, and the treasure you have acquired. And you told me quite a bit about the problems you experienced along the way."

The wise monk paused for a moment to let his words sink in. Then he said,

"Yet, you have not told me...

"Who are you?"

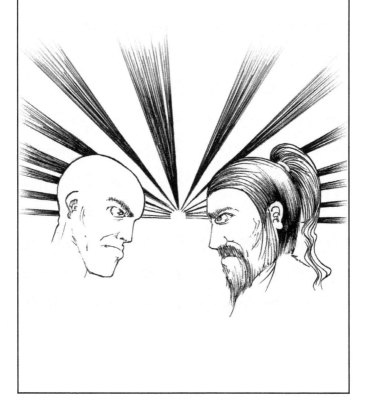

In complete dismay, the young warrior pleaded,

"Please tell me, wise monk, who am I?"

The wise monk then said something most comforting,

"Young warrior, take heart...

You have to be a little cracked to let the light in...

Come, let us take a walk together."

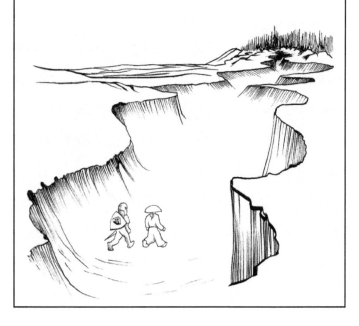

The wise monk led the young warrior along a rolling path through a beautiful valley, deep into the forest. The **smell of the trees,** the **warm sunshine,** and the **joyful sound of nature** soon **calmed** the **friction** within the young warrior's mind.

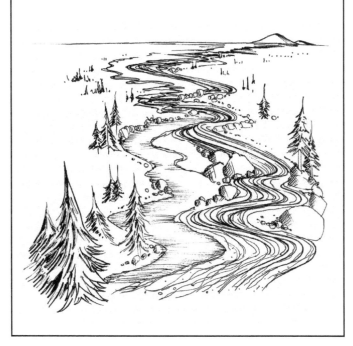

While they walked together, the wise monk offered encouragement to the young warrior.

"I will tell you exactly who you are…" said the wise monk,

"You are a child of God."

Observing the uncertainty on the young warrior's face, the wise monk continued,

"You have been on a quest to find happiness, but happiness is not something you can find…

"Happiness is what you are when you remember who you are."

The wise monk began to explain great spiritual truths in a way the young warrior could fully understand.

"Consider a sunbeam. A sunbeam does not search for the sun, because it's **coming from the sun.**

Or the branch of a vine...

A branch does not search for the vine; the **branch** is already **part of the vine.**[9]

Or a wave of the ocean...

A wave does not look for the ocean; the **wave is from the ocean,** and will therefore also return to the ocean."

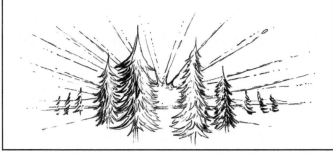

The wise monk looked intently into the eyes of the young warrior, and then continued,

"Because you do not know who you *really are*, you believe all the labels about yourself. To the extent you **believe in the labels** of your life, you **believe in an illusion,** for the labels of your life are **nothing but a story** you tell yourself."

The young warrior objected and said,

"But I think the labels are important to me; they define who I am in the world."

The wise monk explained,

"Your thinking about the labels, just like the material objects of the world, are simply clouds in the sky. They come and go. It is the attachment and aversion to material objects and labels that ultimately cause all the suffering in your life."[10]

The wise monk and young warrior then came upon a beautiful, small pond in the middle of the forest. Leading the young warrior close to the water's edge, the wise monk inquired,

"Can you see your reflection in the water?"

Peering over the edge of the shore, the young warrior noticed his reflection in the stillness of the water.

Unexpectedly, the wise monk threw a large rock into the water, causing a huge splash.

"How about now!" laughed the wise monk.

"Why did you do that? Now the water is too choppy for me to see my reflection," said the young warrior.

The wise monk explained,

"I wanted to give you an example for the nature of your mind. **When your mind is still and clear,** then your **True Source can be reflected back to you,** as if your soul were looking into a polished mirror. However, when your mind is full of turbulence, and all you can see or hear is your own thinking, the mirror becomes filthy, and you can no longer see what you look like."[11]

The wise monk then paused for a moment to ensure the young warrior was listening very closely.

Then the wise monk said something that resurfaced a dormant memory within the young warrior's mind...

"I hope you are beginning to understand that your True Source is God."

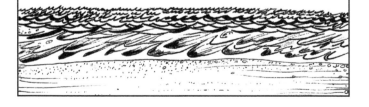

In silence, the young warrior and the wise monk continued their walk through the forest. As they journeyed together, the young warrior reflected on both his triumphs and tragedies. Although it was sometimes very painful, he realized that ultimately he was responsible for every effect of his life.

However, by taking responsibility for the effects of his life, the young warrior felt empowered to pay more attention to their cause, which were his very thoughts.

The young warrior now realized the inner world of his thinking was the ultimate battleground for the true warrior.

The young warrior then asked the wise monk,

"How can I influence the quality of my thinking?"

"This question, young warrior..."

replied the wise monk,

"Is a very good question, indeed."

The wise monk then continued,

"A warrior must be skillful both in action, and non-action.[12]

Action is the world of effects, and non-action is the world of cause. The first step, therefore, is to remove yourself from the world of effects, and to **become still.**"

The young warrior asked,

"Do you mean, I just have to sit down, and stop moving?"

The wise monk laughed and replied,

"Yes! The first step is as simple as that. When the **body becomes still, the mind will surely follow.** I also recommend closing your eyes, which will help turn your **attention inward.** When you focus your attention inward, you are able to **connect with God."** (13)

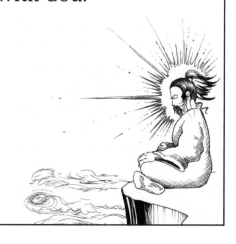

The wise monk then continued to increase the wisdom and knowledge of the young warrior.

"The next step is to become aware of your breathing. The quality of your breathing, the quality of your posture, and the quality of your thinking, are all intimately connected. Bringing your awareness to your breathing, your posture, and your thinking is known as 'mindfulness,' which means to hold your awareness on the present moment and task at hand."

The young warrior asked, "How can I develop awareness of my breath?"

"When you breathe in, know that you are breathing in," answered the wise monk, "And when you breathe out, know that you are breathing out."

Perplexed by this seemingly obvious instruction, the young warrior defensively replied,

"I have been breathing just fine my entire life."

Full of patience, the wise monk explained,

"**Automatic** breathing and **mindful** breathing are worlds apart. In the moments that you are **intensely aware** of the **inhalation** and **exhalation** within a **single breathing cycle**, you become fully alive in the present moment. Although your mind can regress to the past, or project into the future, **your breath** is always **right here, right now** — like an **anchor for your soul.**" [14]

Due to the young warrior's extensive training within the world of action, he was well aware of the significance of respiratory conditioning. The young warrior reflected on moments in his life when his ability to command his breathing while overcoming dragons was absolutely critical to victory.

Full of promise and intrigue, the young warrior exclaimed,

"The power of the breath is something I feel compelled to learn more about. In addition to bringing awareness to every inhalation and exhalation, what else do you recommend I do?"

The wise monk continued to elaborate on the significance of the breath...

"The **inhalation** should be **long, slow, subtle, deep,** and should **evenly spread** throughout the entire body. Each in-breath draws energy from the atmosphere into the cells of the lungs. This **rejuvenates the spiritual force** within you. By **briefly holding** the breath once drawn in, the energy is **fully absorbed.** This evenly distributes it through all the systems of your body.

The **slow** and **peaceful exhalation** removes mental and physical toxins that have been accumulated. **Pause briefly** after the out-breath so that **all mental stress is purged away.** The mind is then naturally drawn into the **presence of God.**"

With a look of awe and wonder on his face, the young warrior remarked,

"I had no idea so much **transformation** could take place within **a single breath!**"

Smiling broadly, the wise monk said,

"Indeed, young warrior, a **daily breath practice** can **enhance** every aspect of your **life.** This is why the ancient Prophets said, '**The breath of God gives life.**'"[15]

The young warrior inquired,

"What constitutes a breath practice?"

The wise monk answered,

"Even **one conscious breath** a day is sufficient to experience all the **benefits of a breath practice.**"[16]

The wise monk then proposed they sit together and experience the power of physical stillness, upright posture, and mindful breathing.

Directing the young warrior to sit with his body, neck, and head held firmly in a straight line with his eyes closed, the wise monk then led him through an ancient breathing practice designed to bring the mind to a state of restful alertness. [17]

The wise monk began by saying...

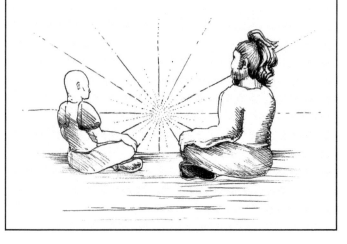

"Be sure to **breathe through your nose** the entire time.

Now **inhale** and count to four....

Retain the breath for another four count....

Exhale for a four count....

Suspend the breath for a four count."[18]

The wise monk and the young warrior continued this breathing sequence for a total of four rounds.

As the breathing practice concluded, a large smile appeared on the young warrior's face.

"I feel wonderful!" exclaimed the young warrior. "I always knew the benefit of **upright posture.** However, I never realized something as simple as **physical stillness** and **mindful breathing** could have such a **profound effect** on me."

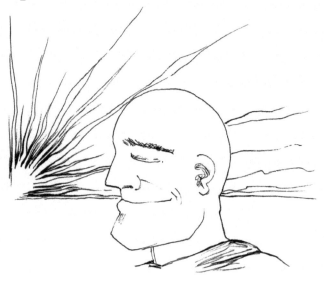

The wise monk nodded in agreement, and replied,

"Because your quest to find God is an inward journey, you will find physical stillness and mindful breathing to be of great benefit to you."

Hearing this, the young warrior asked,

"What do you mean by an 'inward journey?'"

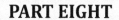

PART EIGHT

MOVING TOWARDS STILLNESS

"The inward journey is a quest to find stillness in the presence of God."

— The Wise Monk

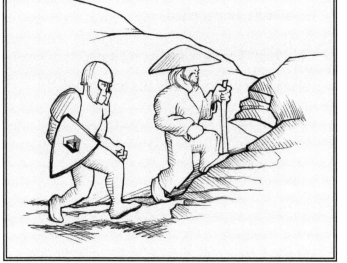

The wise monk then explained a very important spiritual concept for the young warrior to understand...

"Only the inward journey will lead you to the presence of God, and thus true and lasting happiness."

The young warrior clarified,

"Is this why my quest to find happiness through the acquisition of treasure in the world never fully satisfied me?"

The wise monk replied,

"Yes, that is correct. God is not found **out there,"** said the wise monk, pointing to the horizon...

"The presence of God will be discovered in here." The monk continued, pointing to his heart. "Even beneath the conscious level of your thinking."

The young warrior asked in bewilderment,

"What could possibly be beneath my conscious level of thought?"

The wise monk said,

"Beneath your conscious level of thought an abundant reservoir of your True Source awaits. Dipping into this reservoir on a regular and consistent basis will take you places you have never dreamed of."

"I want to go!" the young warrior exclaimed.

"I was so preoccupied with thinking about treasure and dragons, I never realized an **abundant, life-changing reservoir** was available to me," confessed the young warrior.

"You were consumed with treasure and dragons simply because you were thinking about them. You must change the way you think," explained the wise monk.

"Whatever you spend the majority of time thinking about will capture your attention," added the wise monk. "Your attention is like a giant magnifying glass; anything you focus it upon will increase in your life. Similarly, removing your attention from something will cause it to wither and fade away."

"You must penetrate to the very source of thought, which is that part of your being that has direct resonance with God. This is your subconscious mind, and is what the Prophets referred to in their use of the word 'Heart.'"[19a]

"If you recall, I informed you of the magnificent truth:

'As a man thinketh in his heart, so is he.'"[19b]

Nodding in agreement, the young warrior acknowledged his recollection of the wise monk's teaching.

Then the wise monk said something of immense importance…

"Now then, let me share with you an even more profound Truth, spoken by the Great Prophet, which encompasses within it the summing up of the entire pursuit of happiness...

'Blessed are the pure in heart, for they shall see God.'"[20]

Hearing this, a startled expression immediately appeared on the young warrior's face, and he proclaimed,

"You mean to tell me, wise monk, that I will be able to actually see God?"

The wise monk replied with confidence,

"Yes, that is exactly what I am proposing. However, you must understand the Greatest of all Prophets used the word 'See' and 'Heart' in a very special way.

To 'See God' refers to spiritual perception, which means your ability to understand the nature of your true being as a child of God."

The young warrior asked, "Is spiritual perception achieved through my inward journey?"

The wise monk replied,

"That is exactly right! The inward journey is a quest to find stillness in the presence of God. This is why the Great Prophet said that in order to see God, you must first be 'Pure in Heart.'"

The wise monk then continued to teach the young warrior a supremely important lesson...

"When the Great Prophet referred to your 'heart,' he was describing that part of your mentality known as your 'subconscious mind'."

Pausing a moment to ensure the young warrior was listening carefully, the wise monk then continued,

"In other words, young warrior, it is not enough to understand God as your True Source with your conscious mind only. This great truth must also be embraced by your heart. Only then can it circulate throughout your entire being and make a real difference in your character and life."

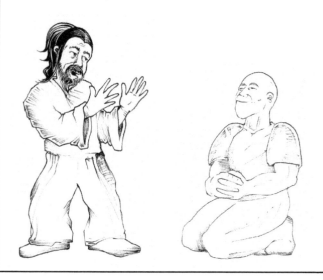

Although the young warrior was listening intently, and doing his very best to understand the magnitude of the wise monk's teaching, this concept proved very challenging for him to comprehend.

The young warrior then posed a question asked universally of all warriors...

"I am desirous of embarking upon the inward journey, yet I feel overwhelmed by the quest set before me. How can I be assured the inward journey will not lead to the same heartache and despair I experienced in my pursuit of worldly treasure?"

The wise monk smiled and nodded with compassion,

"Assurance on the inward journey is a timeless question, for the **path becomes narrow** to those **courageous enough** to **embark** upon this **quest.**[21] However, let me encourage you to understand that only the inward journey will lead you to a pure heart, and allow you to **experience God** as your **True Source** and **True Cause.** In other words, only the inward journey will lead to lasting happiness."

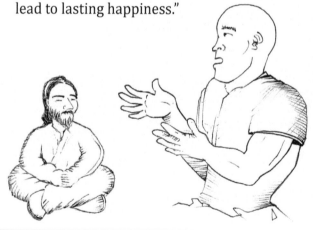

The young warrior then asked,

"Do you think I will be successful on this journey?"

The wise monk replied,

"Yes, of course!

A warrior is supremely suited for the inward journey." [22]

The young warrior smiled at this reassurance.

"Consider this..." the wise monk began,

"As a warrior, you have become skilled in the **domain of action.** Therefore, you have learned that success in physical action is dependent upon moving from **core to extremity.**"

Reflecting for a moment, the young warrior recalled his training in the martial way, and the physical skills he had mastered within the domain of action.

With renewed confidence in himself, the young warrior said,

"Yes, of course! I think I'm beginning to understand the principle involved."

Encouraging the young warrior to elaborate, the wise monk said, "Very good! Tell me more..."

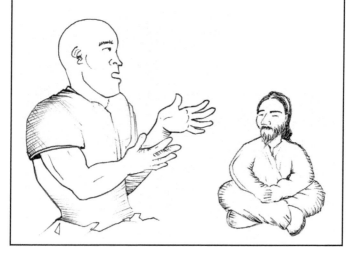

The young warrior explained, "In physical training within the world of *action*, I have learned power is achieved through a contraction of my muscles from my core to extremity."

Nodding in approval, and continuing to build the young warrior's momentum, the wise monk said,

"Yes, this is very good indeed. Now tell me, where is your core?"

The young warrior replied,

"My core is here..." the young warrior said, pointing to his midsection, hips, and low back. "As I engage the large muscles of my hips, they transfer power to the smaller muscles of my extremities."

The wise monk smiled broadly and replied,

"I am very proud of you, young warrior. For the knowledge you have achieved in the world of action may now serve you well in the world of non-action."

The wise monk then explained a very important concept for the young warrior to understand.

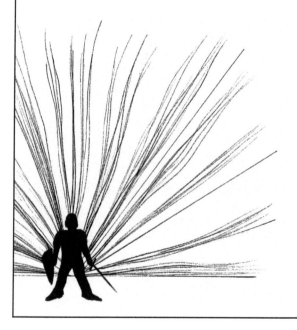

PART NINE

FINDING YOUR TRUE CORE

"God is your True Core, and your True Source, and the True Cause of everything in the entire Universe."

— The Wise Monk

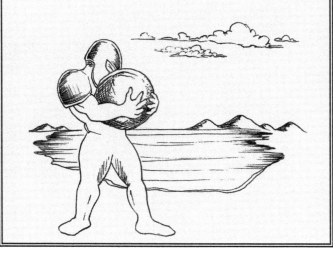

"You see, young warrior, your **True Core** is not the physical one you have mastered in the world of action. Your **True Core** is the **presence of God** within you. **God** is your...

True Core, and your

True Source, and the

True Cause

of everything in the entire Universe." [23]

Because the young warrior knew the significance of his physical core in the world of action, he was able to grasp the lesson the wise monk was now teaching.

The young warrior then asked an important clarifying question,

"Is this what you meant when you said...

'A true warrior must be skillful both in action, and non-action?'"

The wise monk smiled approvingly and said,

"Yes, that is exactly right. Now, follow me, there are two further lessons I wish to share with you."

The wise monk led the warrior deeper into the forest. As they walked along in silence, the young warrior reflected on everything he was learning. He felt grateful for the immense wisdom the wise monk had shared with him, and also a heightened sense of urgency to begin his inward journey.

Because the young warrior had spent so many years in the world of action, and in the pursuit of worldly treasure, he had a tendency to associate his self-worth with the approval of others, and the accomplishment of external reward.

Although he was beginning to understand the greatest treasure of all was within, the young warrior still held reservations that he would be successful upon his quest.

"Wise monk...." the young warrior asked as they continued to walk through the forest,

"Do you really believe I will be able

to **find God,** and connect with my

True Source?"

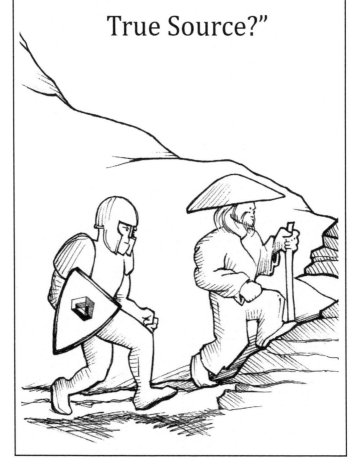

Although he heard the question, the wise monk did not answer, and continued to walk at a brisk pace along the forest path.

The young warrior followed closely behind, and a few moments later, he repeated himself in a slightly louder voice, just to be sure the wise monk heard the question. However, despite his persistence, the wise monk remained silent and continued to press forward, deeper into the forest.

Feeling ignored, the young warrior's internal dialogue became increasingly frustrated and anxious. The young warrior pouted to himself, and wondered if the wise monk would ever answer his question.

And then...

The wise monk abruptly stopped in his tracks, and whispered,

"Young warrior,
listen carefully...
can you hear that sound?"

However, in that moment, the young warrior could only hear the sound of his internal voice, banging between his ears.

"I cannot hear anything except my own thinking!" exclaimed the young warrior.

"Then **become still, close your eyes, and take a long, slow deep breath,**" instructed the wise monk.

Doing as he was told, the young warrior stood very still on the forest path, and closed his eyes. Then he took a long breath in, and a slow breath out. In a few moments, his mind and body began to relax, and he felt a bit more at peace.

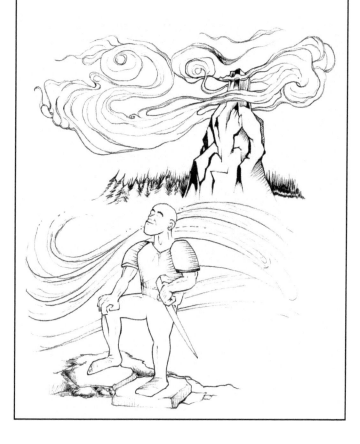

Then, far off in the distance, the young warrior began to detect the sound of moving water. His ears resignated with the unmistakable vibration of a river, rushing against rocks, and moving with the powerful force of nature.

"I can hear the river!" exclaimed the young warrior.

The wise monk replied,

"Find God from there."

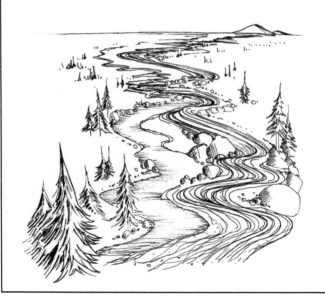

"What do you mean?" questioned the young warrior.

The wise monk answered,

"The sound of the river was there the entire time, only you could not hear it. You first needed to become still, and available to the present moment. This is also how you experience God, for the river of God is always running through you."

The young warrior was elated by the lesson the wise monk had imparted to him.

"Come, let us continue to the source of the river," said the wise monk, who turned and walked further into the forest.

The path twisted and turned through the trees, and then suddenly opened to reveal a majestic lake of deep, blue water. The young warrior thought to himself he had never beheld such a beautiful sight in all his life.

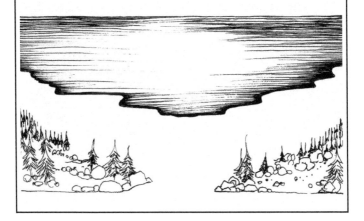

The wise monk led the young warrior to a large pile of massive rocks stacked near the lake.

"Young warrior, pick up one of these rocks and hold it against your chest," the wise monk instructed.

Gladly accepting the challenge and an opportunity to display his strength in the world of action, the young warrior bent down, and hoisted up the largest rock he could find. With his arms wrapped around the rock, he held it firmly against his chest.

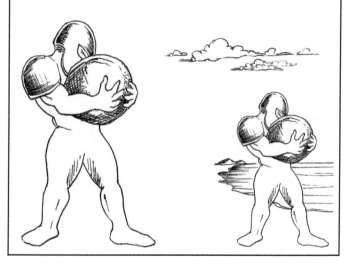

"Very good work, young warrior! You are indeed physically strong. Now, hold that rock at arm's length, directly in front of you," challenged the wise monk.

The young warrior made a valiant effort, but was not able to separate the rock even an inch from his body, for it was far too heavy.

"That's not possible! In order to hold the rock, I must keep it pressed against my body," explained the young warrior.

Looking intently into the eyes of the young warrior, the wise monk said,

"In other words, you must hold the rock close to your core. Is that correct?"

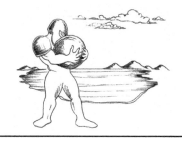

In that moment, the young warrior achieved another moment of increased enlightenment. For in addition to becoming still and silent to fully experience the presence of God, the young warrior now understood the **spiritual significance** of **his True Core.**

Dropping the rock, the young warrior said with great enthusiasm, "Now I understand!"

"I am most capable when I hold external objects close to my core. And similarly, when I turn my attention from the world of action, to the ultimate reservoir of non-action, I experience my greatest strength of all, which is my **True Core.**"

The wise monk nodded in approval, and then posed a question,

"And what is your True Core?"

The young warrior smiled in delight,

"God is my True Core

and therefore my

True Source of strength.

And because

God is within me,

I can share in that strength." [24]

The wise monk once again nodded in approval and admiration of the young warrior's progress.

"Very good, young warrior. You are clearly progressing on the inward journey. There is one final tool I would like to share with you, that will be of immense help in further connecting with your True Source, and in developing a pure heart."

Suddenly, a breeze blew across the lake, and the surface of the water that had been still a moment before, now became very choppy. The wise monk led the young warrior near the water's edge, and together they observed the turbulent conditions of the lake.

The wise monk inquired,

"Young warrior, do you **see how choppy the surface** of the lake is?"

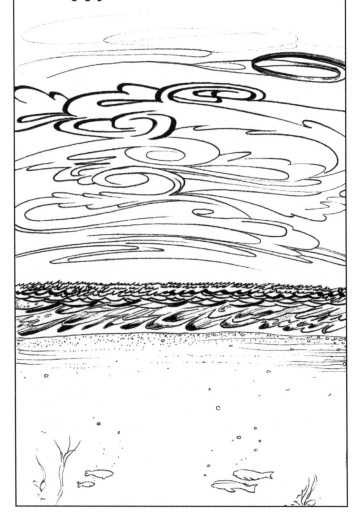

The young warrior nodded in observance of the **storm-like conditions** of the lake's surface.

"Very good..." continued the wise monk. "Now then, consider this: Just a few inches **beneath the surface** of the water, the **choppy conditions** we are now witnessing are a little **bit calmer.**"

As the wise monk continued, the young warrior's eyes displayed an inner comprehension of increasing spiritual knowledge...

"And a **few inches below** that, the conditions are even further removed from the choppiness of the surface. In other words, **each layer beneath** the **surface** becomes a **deeper refuge** of **stillness.**"

The wise monk picked up a rock near the edge of the shore and said,

"Now, imagine if we dropped this rock through the surface of the water, and followed its downward journey to the **very bottom of the lake.** As the rock continued to **sink deeper and deeper** beneath the surface of the water, the **choppiness** and **turbulence** we now observe would be **replaced** by **stillness, peace,** and **quietness.** Ultimately, this rock would come to rest at the very bottom of the lake, where it would sit **motionless,** and **completely undisturbed** by the conditions that once troubled it upon the surface." [25]

The young warrior felt certain this example of the rock and lake was a metaphor for a profound spiritual insight, and he proposed to the wise monk...

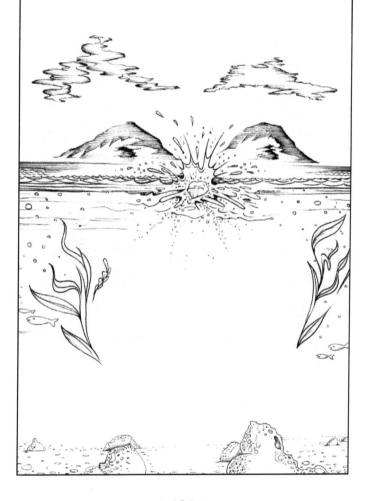

"I believe I understand the lesson you have set before me. The choppy and turbulent conditions at the surface of the lake represent my mind during moments of anxiety, stress and negativity. The bottom of the lake, therefore, is my True Source, the presence of God, where I can sit completely at peace."

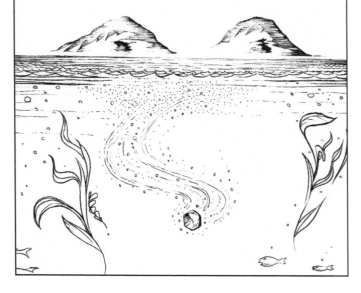

The wise monk smiled, clapped his hands, and exclaimed,

"Yes, that is exactly right! Very good, young warrior."

The young warrior replied,

"However, I do not understand the significance of the rock."

The wise monk then explained his final lesson to the young warrior, a lesson that would prove invaluable along his journey.

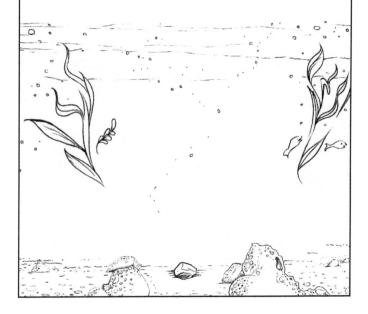

"The metaphor of the rock is the final lesson I wish to share with you. On the inward journey, the repetition of a prayer word within your mind will serve the same effect as the rock within the lake. The repeated prayer word will sink deeper and deeper beneath your conscious level of thinking, which is analogous to the choppy surface of the water. Ultimately, the prayer word will come to rest upon your True Core, the very presence of God within you." [26]

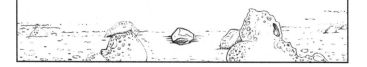

Hearing this, the young warrior was overjoyed. He understood the metaphor the wise monk had taught, and was eager to discover more.

The young warrior then asked an important question,

"Is the repetition of a prayer word within my mind further supported by mindful breathing, and good posture?"

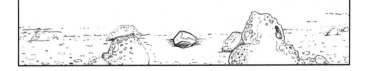

The wise monk smiled with admiration for the young warrior's spiritual progress and answered,

"Young warrior, perhaps one day soon, you will walk the path of a monk, for once again you ask the proper question. The repetition of a **prayer word** within your mind will be **most effective** when you are **seated quietly** with good posture, your **eyes closed,** and your awareness gently placed upon your breathing."

The young warrior then asked,

"And what is the **prayer word**
I shall repeat within my mind?"

The wise monk replied,

"This is, perhaps, the most important question of all. The **prayer word** I recommend you repeat within your mind is the **meaning** of the ancient Hebrew **Name of God,** which is, '**I AM.**'" [27]

"What does, '**I AM**' refer to?" asked the young warrior.

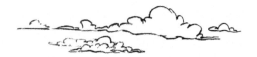

The wise monk explained,

"In the ancient Scriptures, we discover 'I AM' constitutes a most perfect statement for God — the Universal Life that is,

'Over all, and Through all, and In all.'[28]

God is THE ONE True Source, the UNITY of SPIRIT from which all individualities both proceed from and are included within.

When you repeat the prayer word 'I AM' within your conscious mind, you impress upon your subconscious mind your oneness with God, and therefore with everything you may desire. This is why the Great Prophet said...

'Seek God first, and everything else will be added to you.'"[29]

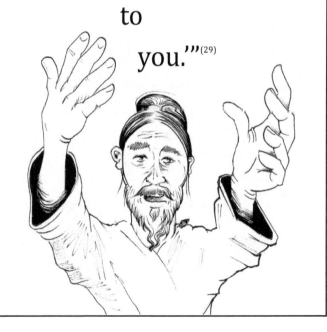

The wise monk then explained how to use the prayer word...

"With your eyes closed and your awareness placed gently upon your breath, begin to repeat, 'I AM' in your mind...

There is no need to strain or force the matter.

Just gently repeat, 'I AM' and trust the sacred meaning of the Name of God will support your intention. In the event you notice yourself thinking anything other than the prayer word, simply become aware of the departure, and then return to your practice of repeating, 'I AM.'"

The young warrior asked,

"How long each day should I engage in this practice?"

The wise monk replied,

"Remember, even a little effort on the path of spiritual progress will serve you well. Perhaps begin with two, ten-minute seated practices a day, and increase in duration from there. I have found the most benefit from two twenty-minute practices, one in the morning upon awakening, and another in the evening."

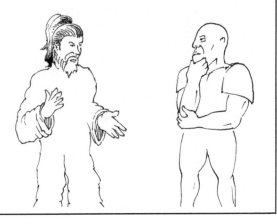

The wise monk humbly bowed to the young warrior, and said,

"I admire your courage to walk the path of a true warrior, both in the world of action, and non-action. Remember these words as you embark onto the next chapter of your life…

'God is more worthy of your pursuit, attention and love than all the other passions of the world combined.'[30]

Furthermore, young warrior, whenever you feel troubled, repeat this affirmation to yourself, either in your mind, or softly whispered out loud...

'God is entirely devoted to my personal advancement.'"[31]

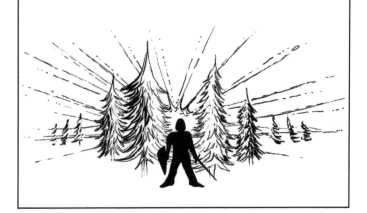

With these profound statements still hanging in the air, the wise monk handed the young warrior a neatly folded letter, then bid him farewell and walked into the forest.

Sensing a great loss and feeling of abandonment, the young warrior objected and said,

"Please don't leave yet!

I have so much more to learn from you."

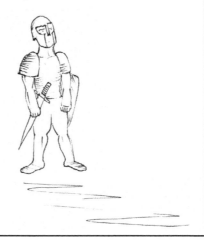

The wise monk turned and looked with **compassion** and **love** into the eyes of the young warrior. He then smiled warmly and said,

"Our paths will soon cross again, **for I have much more to share with you.** The next time we meet, I will tell you of the most marvelous and **greatest news** you have ever heard!"

Overjoyed with expectancy, the young warrior asked,

"And what **great news** is that?"

"Young warrior, what would you think if I told you that **God had a Son**, who became a **Mighty King**, and was the **Greatest Warrior** to have ever lived?" [32]

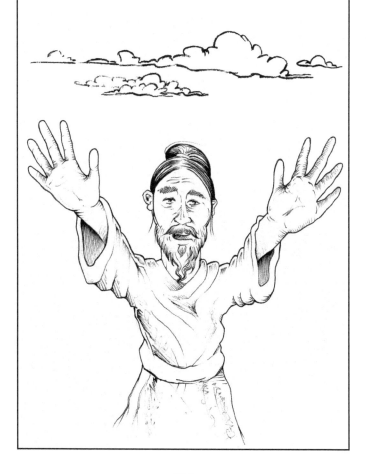

The young warrior stared at the wise monk with a look of astonishment upon his face, and then asked,

"Is this the

Great Prophet

you referred to?"

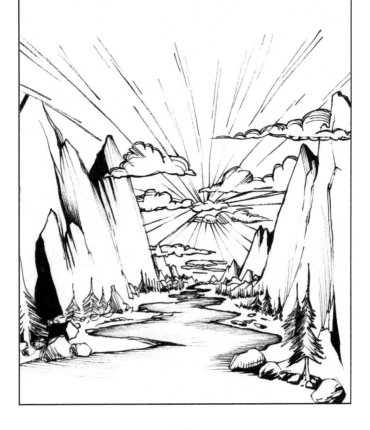

With delight twinkling in his eyes, the wise monk looked over his shoulder as he continued into the forest and said,

"Very well then! Until we meet again...

'May you continue to grow in wisdom, stature and favor with God and mankind.'"[33]

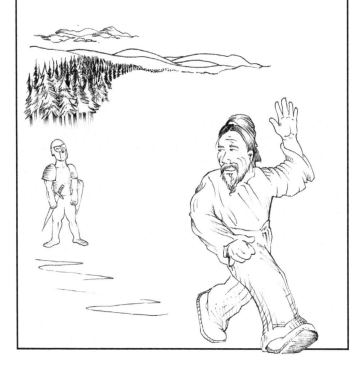

THE SADHANA OF
A TRUE WARRIOR

"A true warrior sets out on a daily
path of self-mastery."

— The Wise Monk

For a few moments, after watching the wise monk disappear into the magnificent forest, the young warrior felt alone.

The impulse to chase after the wise monk nearly overtook him, and he wondered why the monk could possibly leave when he still had so much more to learn.

Standing on the forest path, the young warrior then carefully observed the letter the wise monk had given him. As he gently unfolded the paper and beheld the words written within, a sudden jolt of supernatural energy seemed to rise within him.

The young warrior took a deep breath in, and a slow breath out, and became still in the **presence of a power** he intuitively knew **would now** sustain and **guide his journey.**

The young warrior read aloud the words written in the letter...

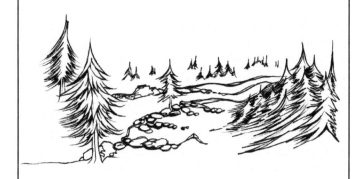

"Young warrior, the ancient spiritual texts collectively instructed the **adherence** to a *Sadhana*, which means 'dedication to daily practice.'

Therefore, I encourage you to **follow very closely** the *Sadhana* outlined here.

Strive daily to master yourself; for in the **disciplined pursuit of self-mastery** you can be of **great service to others.**(34)

Above all, remember that **true happiness** can **only** be achieved through **developing a personal relationship with God.**"

This is your *Sadhana...*

1) Each morning upon awakening, **remain silent.** Begin your day by drinking a large glass of water.

2) Next, go to your **"altar"** or a section of your home you intend to reserve for **communion with God.**

3) **Sit comfortably** with your **body, neck,** and **head** held in a **straight line,** and close your eyes. Then, take four rounds of the **Warrior Breath.**[18]

4) Begin the sacred practice of your **prayer word meditation.** Gradually increase the duration to a comfortable period, between ten and twenty minutes is best.

5) Next, bring into the **temple of your mind** a most perfect statement that expresses the **great heart** within you. **Repeat your affirmation several times.** You may also wish to **repeat ancient Scripture,** or the confirmation, **"God is entirely devoted to my personal advancement."**

6) Now, the practice of **First Words.** Softly break the sacred silence of the morning by **speaking your internally-repeated affirmation out-loud.** Trust the words you speak will **create a rippling effect** through the **ocean** of **God's Universe,** ultimately touching every corner of your life.

7) Spend five to ten minutes studying the ancient spiritual texts. The Holy Bible, Yoga Sutra of Patanjali, and Bhagavad Gita are best. I recommend beginning with the Book of James within the Bible, who was the Greatest Prophet's half-brother.

8) Eat at least three balanced meals a day; a large serving of fruits and vegetables, a fist-sized portion of protein, and a sprinkling of healthy fat is best.

9) Drink between ½ to 1 gallon of fresh water over the course of your day.

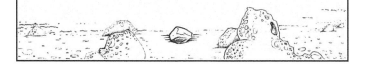

10) **Exercise your body every day.** A combination of Kokoro Yoga or functional gymnastic and weightlifting movements, coupled with variance and an appropriate level of intensity, is best. Whenever possible, take your exercise program outdoors. Spending time in nature will significantly increase the benefit of your practice.

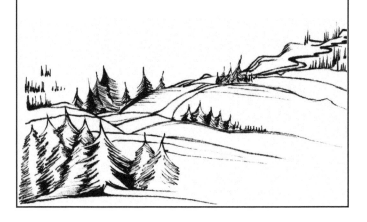

11) Before you retire at night, return to your "altar" or dedicated place of worship. Sit comfortably with your body, neck, and head held in a straight line, and close your eyes. Take four rounds of the Warrior Breath. Then recapitulate your entire day, and contemplate these three questions:

What are you most grateful for?

What is God equipping you for?

How can you best serve others?

"Young warrior, I believe unconditionally in you, and in your ability to succeed. Commit to your *Sadhana*, trust in God, and when you feel ready, teach these principles to all those whom you hold dearly in your life."

— The Wise Monk

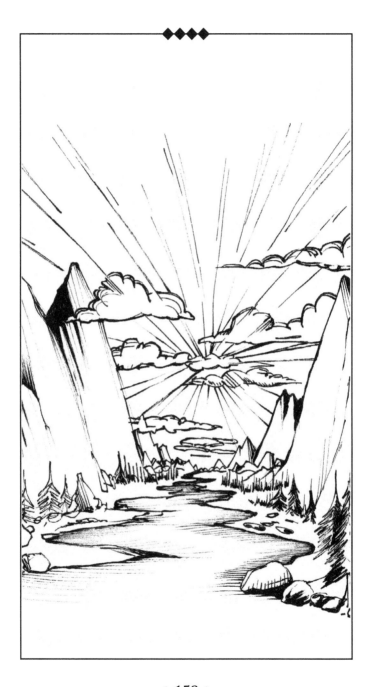

NOTES

(1)   Romans 1:25

(2)   Proverbs 23:7

(3)   Proverbs 4:23

(4)   Deepak Chopra *Seven Spiritual Laws of Success,* New World Library, Amber-Allen Publishing (November 9, 1994)

(5)   Genesis 1:11, Proverbs 18:20-21, Matthew 12:35-37

(6)   2 Samuel 22: 2-3; 31-33

(7)   Luke 17:21

(8)   The Bhagavad Gita 2:40

(9)   John 15:5

(10)   Yoga Sutra of Patanjali 1:15

(11)   James 1:23, Yoga Sutra of Patanjali 1:3-4

(12)   Mark Divine, Navy SEAL Commander (RET.), Founder of SEALFIT and author of *New York Times* best selling book, *Unbeatable Mind* and *Way of the SEAL*

(13)   Yoga Sutra of Patanjali 2:29

(14)   Hebrews 6:19

(15)   Job 33:4

(16)   Dan Brulé, World renowned breathwork pioneer and author of the book, *Just Breathe*

(17)   The Bhagavad Gita 6:13

(18)   The Four Count Breathing Exercise is refered to as "Box Breathing" or "Warrior Breath"

(19a)   Walter A. Elwell, *Evangelical Dictionary of Theology,* Baker Academic; 3rd Edition (November 7, 2017)

(19b)   Proverbs 23:7

(20)   Matthew 5:8

(21)   Matthew 7:13

(22)   The Bhagavad Gita 2:31

(23)   Genesis 1:31

(24)   Isaiah 40:29, Philippians 4:13

(25)   Yoga Sutra of Patanjali 1:2

(26)   Hebrews 4:9-13

(27)   Exodus 3:14 — God's name is almost always translated LORD (all uppercase) in the English Bible. But the ancient Hebrew name for God would be pronounced "YAHWEH," and is built on the Hebrew word for "I AM THAT I AM." Therefore, the word "YAHWEH" may be substituted for "I AM" as the meditative prayer word. Additional training on mantra meditation is available at www.TM.org

(28)   Ephesians 4:6

(29)   Matthew 6:33

(30)   Raymond Amundson

(31)   Julianne Amundson

(32)   John 3:16, Revelation 19:11-16

(33)   Luke 2:52

(34)   Yoga Sutra of Patanjali 2:1

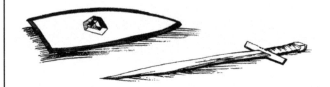

ALSO FROM BEST SELLING AUTHOR
GREG AMUNDSON

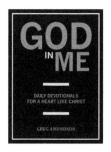

In a unique and powerful new voice, Greg Amundson merges Biblical truth with modern day lessons on leadership, positive thinking, and the warrior spirit. Each day of the year, you will be guided scripturally through the key principles and teachings from the Bible, resulting in a more intimate relationship with God and understanding of His Word.

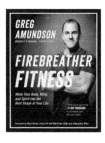

Greg Amundson's effective guides to functional fitness, nutrition, goal-setting, pain tolerance, honing purpose and focus, and exerting control over your mental state are designed to help meet any challenge. Packed with practical advice, vetted training methods, and Amundson's guided workout programs, *Firebreather Fitness* is a must-have resource for athletes, coaches, law enforcement and military professionals, and anyone interested in pursuing the high-performance life. Includes a foreword from *New York Times* bestselling author Mark Divine.

ALSO FROM BESTSELLING AUTHOR
JOE DE SENA

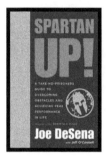

Spartan Up! A Take-No-Prisoners Guide to Overcoming Obstacles and Achieving Peak Performance in Life. Spartan founder, Joe De Sena, leads the way in an inspirational book on how to achieve peak performance in every area of your life.

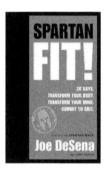

Spartan Fit! 30 Days. Transform Your Mind. Transform Your Body. Commit to Grit. Joe De Sena designed the Spartan races to test overall conditioning: strength, flexibility, endurance, and speed. His signature take-no-prisoners approach to achieving physical and mental fitness has taken the endurance world by storm and inspired millions.

COMING IN FALL OF 2018: *The Spartan Way: Eat Better. Train Better. Live Better. Be Better.*

KEYNOTES AND SEMINARS

Greg Amundson is one of North America's most electric, encouraging, and motivating professional speakers. Greg has logged more than 10,000 hours of dynamic public speaking on topics including leadership, intrinsic motivation, holistic 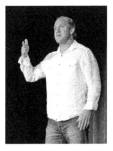 wellness practices, functional fitness, warrior spirit, and God's Love. Greg speaks around the Country to Law Enforcement Departments on integrating disciplined warrior practices to foster increased Officer Safety while simultaneously generating stronger community relationships. A plank owner of the highly regarded Eagle Rise Speaker Bureau, Greg is renowned for his ability to transcend boundaries and speak to the heart of Spirituality. His use of captivating storytelling results in a profound and transformational learning experience.

To book Greg Amundson at your next conference or in-house event please visit www.GregoryAmundson.com.

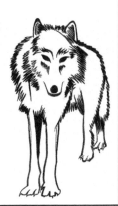

CPSIA information can be obtained
at www.ICGtesting.com
Printed in the USA
BVHW030442280319
543874BV00003B/335/P

9 781611 702729